My Own Eyes

Georjean Privette

Copyright © 2023

All Rights Reserved

Contents

Chapter 01 1

Chapter 02 13

Chapter 03 The Shots 23

Chapter 04 66

Chapter 01

When I was younger, around 7, I wanted to help babies come into the world. I loved, and still do, love babies and the miracle of birth. When I was 18, I became a CNA in the prep for nursing school. In that early phase of my healthcare career, I learned things about human life and interactions. I grew up in the American foster care system, was bounced around a lot, and never knew how the true American family worked. I got married very young, but after having three children and a failing marriage because of adultery, my adult relationships didn't teach me what being a CNA had. As a CNA, I started where every CNA does, in the elderly population at nursing homes. I learned how to love through healthcare. I learned how to interact with older individuals who had lived impressive and some not-so-amazing lives. I loved listening to their stories of family, love, and what they had learned in their lifetimes.

As a CNA, I worked for an agency that placed me in different facilities in Arizona. Living in Tucson, I was close to the border of Mexico and close to many Indian reservations. I worked at a facility about two hours away at one point. I would take my 3 kids to a babysitter (my foster mom I still knew from when I was 12 and placed with her) and would work 16-hour shifts and sleep 8 hours between at a provided apartment on the facility grounds. So I would drop my kids off and drive there on Friday; I would work 3 pm-7 am, sleep, work 3 pm-7a Saturday and then go home to get my kids. When I worked here, I realized the difference in culture between Americans, the Tohono O'odham culture, "T.O." for short.

Usually, when you walk into a 'nursing home,' you get the familiar scent of old urine, cleaning supplies, and milk. I know, weird combo! When you walked into this place, it smelled clean. Not bleach, not cleaning products, just clean. The people that took care of the residents there were all T.O. No one spoke excellent English. I was the lone white person. It was how I got the nickname "milka," which I took as a white person; not sure if that's true. But these were the nicest people and took care of their elders; it was full of respect and dignity. It was a lesson I learned hands-on about what tradition was, what family meant, and how care for your elders should be upheld. This incredible experience has carried me into a nursing career full of respect and acknowledgment of some American culture and healthcare system failures.

I went to nursing school in 2008; It was a challenging but great experience. I still thought I wanted to become a midwife and help babies come into the world. I focused on this and did my last semester training on a labor and delivery floor. This was, again, a life-changing and eye-opening experience. Because I grew up in the system, I had always steered clear of drugs. I knew what they did to individuals, children, and families. It was eye-opening when I would speak to a mother about giving birth who had just smoked marijuana. Don't get me wrong, I am not a prude, marijuana I know it is natural, and I can tell you, in 20 years in healthcare, I have never seen death or overdose from it. However, it's still not suitable for a developing fetus. I also ran into many moms that did more than that, cocaine and opiates. To see these babies born, some left by their moms and taken by the system. However, before the system could take them, we as nurses had to wean them from their addiction created in the womb. It was heartbreaking to see an infant shake and scream (a very high-pitched distinct sound).

One newborn I will never forget, this was not an addicted baby, but a baby that the parents knew would die at birth. She had a lot of malformations, and her brain was not developed. This mom still decided to carry her and let God decide. When she was born, she only lasted a few minutes before God took her home. But this was an amazing sight. As I cleaned her up and wrapped her in a blanket for her parents to hold, her face was perfect to our standards no, but to God. She had smooth sweet skin and one nostril on her nose; it was so weird to be so beautiful with such an odd deformity. Her little lips were heart-shaped. She wasn't born like many infants, with red skin and veins you could see. She looked like a porcelain doll wrapped in a pink blanket given to God as a gift. It opened my eyes to the thought that science and DNA sometimes mess up, but God does not.

When I graduated from nursing school, I still had the thought in my mind that I was going to be a midwife. I was scared and excited when I applied for my first nursing job. I applied it everywhere and then got my first call. It was a bustling emergency department, and I was scared. I had always studied more intensely on birth and pregnancy, and I almost felt I was not smart enough for this. The childhood I had experienced, however, makes me the type of person to know that I can handle anything. I also feel like God has always shown me the way, and through my stubbornness has slowed my path, I always end up where I am supposed to be. I was shopping and driving through town the day before my interview. Now a joke among seasoned nurses is if I am not clocked in, I am not a nurse. But being a new nurse with just school behind me, I was always eager to see if I could help. Right before me, a car hit a man on a motorcycle at a stoplight. He slid on the ground and ended up in the driveway of a business. Of course, I parked my car and jumped out to see if he was ok. I asked him the usual questions to see if he was alert. I slowly helped him lift his helmet off and saw he had two black eyes starting to emerge. I made him lay still and kept asking him questions until EMS arrived. I told them what happened and how he presented and was sure he had a basilar skull fracture. Of course, the EMS crew looked at me, rolled their eyes, and focused on the patient and getting him to the ambulance. But I felt proud of my assessment, I thought that I could handle emergencies, I felt that God again placed me there to show me he knew what I needed to see to have confidence. I used this story in my interview, and I was hired on the spot and started my new job the following week.

The emergency room was full of craziness; I had nightmares during my first six months of nursing. It was intense. I had gunshot wounds, I had septic patients, I had crazy patients, and I even had people that shouldn't be in the ER. Some lessons I learned in my first 5 years in my first job. I remember one night it was nuts; we were so busy, as usual. When traumas or codes come in, each area takes turns. Each site had its doc and code nurse that had to go to the trauma room and complete the code. On this particular night, a code blue came in. It was our area's turn, so my doctor and another nurse went while the third nurse and I stayed in the room to take care of the patients. There was screaming going on, and the code was very long. A call bell went off, I went into the room, and the patient was furious. She said, "I need to see the doctor right now," I said, "Ma'am, I am so sorry you are waiting our doctor is in a code right now." This lady screamed at me, "I don't care, I was here first," astonished. I said, "Ma'am, he is saving someone's life right now." She again yelled at me, "well, get someone else." I asked, "Ma'am, what are you here for?". She responds, "I have a sore throat, and it's killing me." I learned that every patient is not an emergency; some people do not care about others' lives, and that is why EMS and emergency room nurses have the eye roll to an art. However, I already had that growing up; my biggest fault as a kid was a big attitude. Well, it showed that night I responded to this patient, "your sore throat wouldn't hurt if you didn't yell so much" she may have left against medical advice that night, and I may have felt just a little bad, but in the scheme of life, I felt that she didn't need to be there anyways.

As I grew into a better nurse and my skills and confidence grew, I gained respect as a nurse. This turned in to being a charge nurse and preceptor. Now, most times, I truly enjoyed these roles; they made me feel good and taught me as I taught others. To this day, and this was 12 years ago now, I still get random texts from some of the nurses I taught. It's a great feeling to know you made a positive impact. Well, I didn't always make this positive impact, unfortunately. Remember that stubbornness and attitude I talked about? One night I was given a new nurse to precept. She was a bachelor's degree RN; I only had my associate's. So I guess you could say she thought she was a little better. Anyways, It was a wild night.

We were in the busiest area and had very sick patients. It was probably about four hours into the shift, and she walked up to me. She asks, "where are the techs." I said, "I have no clue; why?" She responded, "the patient in that room needs the bedpan," I said, "so go help them with the bedpan." She looked at me like I had two heads and said, "I am a nurse with a bachelor's degree," I said, "I don't care who the hell you are; you are their nurse and need to go help them now." I am always of the opinion that nurses started as CNAs and are far better. It doesn't matter how high you are on the food chain or, in that moment, how high of a nurse you are; you are there to help a patient no matter what they need. About two hours later, one of our patients coded. As we all ran in to start CPR and run this code, this bachelor's prepared nurse was nowhere to be found. After about 30min, the code was done, and the patient was intubated; I decided to speak with her. I asked her where she had been, and she said she had gotten scared; I may have raised my voice some. I responded, "if you can't help with a bedpan, and you can't help save a life, you better get out of here now. You gotta buck up or leave". She left that night crying and upset with me for being stern and not coddling her. However, I understand it is hard. I had nightmares for six long months, but I never once said no to helping a patient, and I never once backed down from a scary life-saving moment, and if you do, I don't care what that college paper says; you are a terrible nurse.

After five years at my first job, I felt I needed to learn and grow. This was when I started traveling. I also started to obtain my bachelor's degree in nursing. I wanted to grow, not for the piece of paper or bragging rights. I felt God had placed it on my heart, and If he did, it would work. I was again a single parent of now 4 children, a new travel nurse, and going to school online. So if it wasn't God's plan, I don't think I would have achieved it. Though I had a great educational start in nursing, you always learn more from a new place, new ways of doing things, and new ways of projecting your experience.

In my first assignment, I learned how to advocate for myself, other nurses, and patients. I was only two weeks into my first contract, and it was a busy day. I had a patient come in that was septic. I knew from my experience that when you have a septic patient, your goals are cultures, fluids, and antibiotics. So, I got my two IVs, started fluids in both, sent off the blood and cultures, and waited for the orders for antibiotics to come through. As I refreshed the screen, I saw an order I wasn't expecting. It was an order for Cardizem bolus and infusion. Cardizem is a medication used to slow down your heart rate if you are in specific rhythms and your blood pressure. Because he was septic, my patient had a heart rate in the 140s, and his blood pressure was low. So I was baffled; I did not know these doctors yet and didn't have to repour with them. I have a rule I follow; if I am unsure of an order, I always go for education first. Maybe I am wrong, perhaps I don't know the reason, and the order makes sense. So I went to the doctor who ordered it. I asked why he had ordered Cardizem, and I was unsure about it. He responded, "well, I am not sure if this is AFIB or SVT, so I want to slow his heart rate down." I replied, "well, sir, the rate is 144, and it is sinus tach, so it's not either of those." I then said, "his blood

My Own Eyes

pressure is also 84 systolic". He looked at me, obviously annoyed, and said, "go get a manual BP," so I did. I returned after that and said, " sir, it's 86 over 54. He looked at me again and said, ok, give 2.5mg until the heart rate comes down. I again did not disagree. I got the patient's vitals again, made many notes, and then went to the charge nurse. UGH, I was sure about to lose my contract; that is what I thought. But I had to do what I thought was right for the patient. So I walked up to the charge nurse, who I didn't know yet, and said, "the doctor wants me to give Cardizem to this guy. He appears septic; I have fluids going, and his blood pressure is still low. I have charted his vitals a few times and made notes. You can read all that and do it if you want. Still, I am refusing this order". She looked at the chart, and because she knew the doc, she yelled to him, "hey doc, why do you want to give Cardizem to this guy: he responded, very annoyed now, "there are studies that say you can give 2.5mg every 5 minutes and it will lower the heart rate". She looked at me, did the famous ER eye roll, and said, "let's move the patient into a room and wait." So we moved him; he didn't get the Cardizem, he got antibiotics, and his heart rate slowly came down after lots of fluids. I learned that day that as a nurse, you sometimes had to throw the fear of losing "your moment's job" in exchange for the life of a patient. As simple as that.

Another lesson I learned was how to advocate for patients and families. Now, the first job I had, was mainly an adult ER. I had treated kids, but it was seldom. Well, this ER was different. It was kids and adults. The first pediatric (kid) trauma I had was not easily forgotten. It was a 14-year-old that was jet skiing and hit a piling. He was showing signs of head trauma. We got him in the room, his blood pressure was elevated from pain, and he was acting forgetful. After a scan of his head showed no brain trauma, the scan of his chest came back. This poor kiddo had an Aortic tear.

There was a tear in the lining of his heart. I had to start him on Esmolol. This medication controls your heart rate and lowers your blood pressure. So I was scared; I had done this before but on an adult. It is so different with a child. I started it, and his blood pressure dropped. Not a lot, but it fell. I got scared and stopped it. When I called to give report to the nurse in intensive care, he laughed and said, "it's supposed to do that; turn it back on." So I did, learning that I was wrong, and monitored him upstairs. The next day, I went upstairs to check on him and his family. I talked to his mom and dad; they were frustrated because he needed surgery, and no specialist there could do it. I told them about a hospital with pediatric surgeons specializing in this type of thing. I got the house supervisor, and we arranged for him to be flown to this other hospital to get surgery. This was a lesson that would serve me very well. Advocacy is so important in healthcare; it's even more critical when health professionals are not doing what is suitable for the patient.

After this travel assignment, I finished my bachelor's degree and traveled to other places. I went to different hospitals; I even did an assignment at a prison (not my thing). But everywhere I went, I learned. I always kept my mind and heart open. I became an advocate for myself, my patients, and other nurses. I started my own business after getting my bachelor's degree. I felt that advocacy was essential but just as important as accountability. I started working for a lawyer doing nurse case reviews. This not only opened my eyes to how the system, healthcare in particular, was also dangerous if you don't know what is going on as a patient or have medical professionals that do not act in the best interest of their patients. This also made me a better nurse. I was able to articulate better when there was an issue. I could chart a patient assessment and story better, so if anything was wrong, there was a clear picture. I also learned that nurses are not governed by the doctors they are under. As a nurse, you are a professional responsible for taking care of your patient and giving them the best and most appropriate care. Sometimes I question an order, sometimes, I am right, and sometimes I am wrong. But I am smart enough to accept that I can be wrong, and others can be too. I also am respectful; I try to be when confronting a doctor or other healthcare professional. I also learned, and try to teach new nurses, that doctors respond better when you have the knowledge to back up your defense. This means don't question something unless you can articulate why it's wrong, what can happen, and other avenues to try.

This aspect of nursing I have slowly gained and perfected ~~this~~. After traveling and being in the float pool, I worked in every hospital area (except labor and delivery) and became an educator and supervisor. I enjoyed this job. I worked with a manager I loved, and I was free to advocate for nurses and patients at this job because I knew and was respected by most of the staff at the healthcare facility. During this time, I also decided I needed to grow more, so I started towards my Masters's degree in nursing education. So again, I started back to school while raising 5 kids and working as an educator. This was when things seemed like they were going great, and I was where God wanted me to be when things went downhill. I would say not for me, but for healthcare, but it has thrown me into a whole new era of my life, and my eyes have opened; this is the story of what I have seen with My Own Eyes.

Chapter 02

When COVID-19 erupted, I, of course, like everyone, was a little scared, but do what I always did. I jump into action, and I educate myself and others. So, I did; I got shields, donated hard hats, and made face shields for the nurses; I handed them out to the staff at the hospital and continued to learn. Then we realized we had shut down all our services and didn't have the COVID craziness they said would come. Instead, the hospital went into the red financially, and we had meetings every day that seemed not to be helping. This was when I had to step down from my position and start working the floor, the hospital didn't have enough money to pay for my place anymore, and we had no staff.

We started getting COVID patients; our county had the first death arise. This patient was about 300lb and refused intubation. He walked into the facility with an oxygen level of 60. He got transferred out and died from a stroke related to COVID. I thought this was the beginning of a horrible virus showing its face. Now working on the floor, we had separated it and closed off a back section to make a "covid" area. It had six beds and started to fill up.

One of the first patients we had with Covid was an elderly lady. She was in her eighties and had been sent from a local nursing facility. The first day she was there, she was pretty sick. She had high fevers and was hallucinating, and we supported her and thought she would get worse. Over the next week, she slowly improved. She was blind from childhood, but she was a spry one. She started eating again; she started acting fine. So we decided she could get out of the hospital. At the beginning of Covid, we had to test people and get two negative results before they could return to the facility they had come from. So we tested her, and at week two, she still tested positive. She was acting fine, so this was a dead virus still in her passageways, but that didn't matter; she had to stay in the hospital. This woman was tested approximately 10 times over the next two months until she finally tested negative. She had multiple positive tests while she was no longer sick. It made me realize I needed to learn more about this virus.

Another patient I remember when all this started was a lady in her mid-forties. She came in from the er and was on 2 liters of oxygen. For my 12 hours with her, I had to increase this to 15 liters. I was very worried about her. I thought for sure she would decline more. We put the cover over her bed and rushed her to the ICU. She was so scared and very alone. I called her husband and told him all that was happening. I reassured him that we were doing all we could. I went and saw this woman every day in the ICU. I checked on her the first day, and she had thrown up. No one had cleaned her or helped her. She felt horrible and now had thrown up in her beautiful long hair. I went in and cleaned her. She could barely move, but she could get into the chair; I washed her hair, brushed it, cleaned her up, and changed her bed. And then saw her smile. Through the fear and struggle, I was able to help her feel like herself again and smile. Even if, for a second, this poor woman had a reprieve from fear and was thankful. I went and repeated this for several days; the staff rolled their eyes when I would walk in and say I was doing too much. I would explain that I would want to come if this were my family or me. It was a familiar face that she had started relying on. This was the same time I decided to leave this hospital, but I discovered that she made it back to the floor, out of ICU, and survived. I thank God for that experience and that he placed me there to help her through that time.

That is when I decided to leave this hospital and educate myself more. I took a staff development position at a facility they were turning into 100 percent COVID-positive nursing home residents. So, we got nursing home residents from all over the state. I educated staff on PPE, respiratory status, and infection control. I saw that these patients were given blood thinners as needed with examining labs because their DDimers were consistently elevated and vitamins helped fight the virus. We had a 94-96 percent survival rate. This was in a facility with an average age of 75, and they appeared to be doing well. Some did not even show symptoms. They were tested on day 21, which gave them 3 weeks of quarantine at our facility. Some continued to test positive and could not return to their facility; however, they maintained their status with their health.

I realized Covid wasn't as scary as it was played out to be.

This realization does not mean that I took this virus lightly. I still was unsure about everything. At this facility, they made me test every employee once weekly, including myself. I did this and rarely got a positive result. I never tested positive while working there. There were a few that tested positive but had no clue. This reminded me of the elderly lady that tested positive for months. So to me, the testing was absurd. When they did PCR testing, I realized they could make one virus particle, dead or alive, expounded to make a positive test. It was, to me, just a way of dotting I's and crossing T's. But I went along with it because I was hired for this.

Fast forward to December 2020. This was when they started giving COVID shots to staff and patients. It was optional then, and I kept my opinions to myself but opted out. I didn't trust this; I hadn't researched it for myself. Some staff members that got it, because I had formed trusting relationships with them, were mad I had not told them not to get this shot. I felt this wasn't my job; I didn't know the effects of it. They were upset; I remember one saying, "if I had known you were not getting it, I wouldn't have" this made me feel bad, but I couldn't tell people what to do, and I could not educate them about what I was still unsure of.

There was a nurse I hired while working there, she joined me for infection control. She was a wise, beautiful woman, and we immediately hit it off because we were both trying to obtain our master's degrees. She was one of the first in line when the shots came out. After I left this job, she called me maybe two months later. She ended up having an enormous cyst on her ovary they thought was cancer. She had to have emergency surgery and a biopsy. It was not cancer, thank god, but was, now I know, a direct result of the covid shot.

I remember one staff member; she was one of my favorites. We always joked around, and she was a great hard worker. She was the first in line to get her covid shot. About two hours after her shot, she sat in a chair in front of me; she didn't look good. I asked her what was wrong; she said things were spinning, and she wasn't sure. She looked terrified and confused. I took her vitals; her blood pressure was 190/100s. She didn't have a history of this. We called her family and sent her to the ER. She stayed there and was given IV meds to reduce her BP. From that day out, she didn't come back to work. I was unable to reach her. I don't know what happened, but I know she lived, but at what cost? Looking back, I now realize this shot is making blood pressure skyrocket.

During this time, while I worked at the COVID facility, my oldest daughter worked at Walmart. I begged her to wear an N95; I didn't know everything about COVID, but I did know it was airborne, and that was the only mask to help. My oldest is a rebel; she does what most liberals do. She virtue signaled with her cute cloth masks and went about her day. Now I love my daughter, even with her own choices and craziness. Well, One day, I came home, and she said, "mom, everything hurts," I said go to bed and sleep; we will see how you feel tomorrow.

The next day I went to work; I came home early and said I would take her to get tested. On the way to the truck, my daughter said, "my chest hurts" my heart immediately sank. But knowing what I did, I took her to the ED. She was tested for COVID, which was negative; I knew they were wrong, but I didn't care; it meant I could be with her. Her troponin and the cardiac enzyme was elevated. Normal is less than 0.03; hers was 0.07. This wasn't huge, but it was elevated in a 20-year-old with chest pain. They admitted her for observation. They released her the next day. I made her lie down as soon as we got home, her heart rate was in the 160s, and she was short of breath. I knew this wasn't the last of it.

The next day I was getting ready, and she begged me to help her with a bath. I filled the tub lukewarm because I felt she needed to be careful with heat. As she was getting out, I was helping her dry off. She looked at me and said, mom, I don't feel well; something is wrong. Right in front of me, my daughter dropped. She fell to the floor, and I screamed. I didn't feel her pulse; she was unconscious. I yelled for my husband to call 911. I got her flat on the floor and had my hands on her chest. Being an ER nurse, it came naturally, but being a mom, I was torn up. She jerked a little, and I felt a pulse again; she had one. Slightly, my hearing returned; I heard my 12-year-old screaming, my husband on the phone, and my seven-year-old crying. And then I listened to the fire rescue men walk in. I hovered over my naked 20-year-old crying; her eyes slowly opened, and I was explaining to fire rescue what had happened. I covered my daughter with a towel and picked her up onto the stretcher.

As they took her to the ambulance, I got her some clothes and rushed to my truck to follow her to the hospital. I was shaking. I got in the truck I couldn't focus. I called my friend to talk to me while I drove. I was screaming and bawling. It was a moment I will never forget. When I pulled up to the ER, I ran in; I was made to put on a mask and wait in the waiting room; it was the longest five minutes. Then they let me back to her room.

When we got to the hospital, the doctor came in, and we told her what had happened. She did blood work and tests, her troponin now was 0.17, and her CT showed opacities in her lungs and fluid around her heart. I said I am sure this is COVID and its pericarditis from it. The cardiologist did not agree; the hospitalist wanted to discharge her. I refused this and asked for an ECHO. She was admitted, then the nurse on the floor came in and said, oh, they want to put her on COVID protocol, and that means... I cut her off.

See, I had worked in a hospital when this started. I saw people alone, not having family, and being scared; I wasn't leaving.

I said. I told them from day one what this was, and they ignored me until I almost did CPR on my child. You will have to get security to remove me. They stopped the COVID protocol, she got her echo and diagnosis of pericarditis, pleural effusion, and viral PNA, and they started colchicine, aspirin, and Motrin. She followed up with a month of bed rest.

I add this about my daughter to the story because it was traumatic and shows what COVID can do when you don't have the proper treatment early. I didn't know about ivermectin then; I didn't know about the early treatment I could have provided for my daughter. I was educated and DID NOT know. I also add this to my story because my daughter, after she healed and wanted to go to college, they required the COVID shot. I begged her not to get it and told her there were side effects. She again didn't listen. She got the johnson and johnson shot. She thought one and done. I cried. She got the shot in mid-2021 in Nov 2021. My daughter texted me, "what does it mean when I can't walk to the bathroom without getting short of breath" I told her, " You need to go to the hospital. Go to the nearest one, and I will meet you there.

When I got there, they called her back. I told the ER nurse that she has pericarditis from her history and the j and j. He said, "ya, I have seen a lot" he continued to say, "when I first saw my first 17-year-old STEMI (which is a heart attack), I knew something was wrong". After some blood work, my daughter's DIMER was 892;

the average is less than 0.5. She got a CT to look for blood clots; it was negative for PE. The doctor then came in and said, we will walk her around and see how she does. I again said she had pericarditis and is now micro-clotting from the shot. He laughed at me and said, no, it's probably fine. So we walked her, and her heart rate went to the 150s, and her O2 went to 92%.

I again refused for her to be discharged and for her to see cardiology and get an echo. So we did, and she did. The echo showed another pleural effusion, pericarditis, and she was to see cardiology and pulmonology for follow-up. She was placed on a colchicine course again, longer this time. Motrin and I put her on vitamins and Nattokinase, a natural blood thinner. She is doing much better today but has worse anxiety; she is scared to get sick, hasn't taken a hot shower since she collapsed, and is not back to her usual physical activities.

I speak this story of my daughter because I should have treated her early with Ivermectin and vitamins. When I knew about them, my husband got COVID, and he was fine in a day with Ivermectin; when I got it (I will tell how I got it), I took ivermectin and had to do doxycycline, zpack, and prednisone because I masked at work, so I was a little worse. My youngest two got it; I increased their vitamins, used homemade quinine, and included quercetin and zinc. I feel bad because my oldest suffered at the hands of the health care she got, and I failed her too. I should have known, but I was not educated when she got sick. This is why I keep pushing to educate others and not allow another young, healthy person to fall because our health system is controlled by noncritical-thinking individuals that refuse to learn.

Now when I got COVID, I was working as a travel nurse. Now you remember, I worked in a hospital when it started and in a 100 percent COVID-positive facility and never got sick. I got COVID from shedding from the shots being given. I work in a small mountain facility; thank god it's a low-vaccination area. However, I still saw the horrible effects of this shot. Even though every time I say it, I get crazy looks from healthcare providers and patients; I will continue the fight to educate.

Chapter 03
The Shots

I had a patient with increased seizures; she had a history of seizures but had not had one for years until she got Moderna. She said, "as soon as I got it, I had a seizure that night" She then said she had 5-6 seizures a day since the shot. The doctor said, "geez, she's crazy, huh." When I went to discharge her, she was crying. I sat down and said, this is real. I believe you. You need to report it to VAERs and call Moderna and report it. She said thank you. She wrote down the information and walked out. When I cleaned her room after she left, I was shocked. I don't mean surprised; the metal bed frame shocked me, and it hurt. I had to walk out without finishing. Since that day, the static electricity while cleaning rooms after patients leave has been constant.

It was a long night, and we were busy with critical patients. A couple came in; the boyfriend was carrying the girlfriend. He said, "we were gonna go on a trip, but she just wasn't acting right and wouldn't wake up" This woman was not alert; she was breathing but appeared very sick. The rapid COVID was positive; she was in septic shock from COVID. We had to intubate her and put her on medications for her blood pressure and sepsis. The boyfriend was sitting on a chair in the hallway crying; I sat down next to him and put my hand on his shoulder. He said, "how is it possible that she has this" "they paid her 100 dollars last week to get the shot". I said what? He said the health department paid people 100 dollars to get the COVID shot, so she can't have it. I kept my hand on his shoulder and let him cry; inside, I was boiling. She was on many medications to sedate her and keep her blood pressure up. I am unsure if she lived or died because we transferred her to another hospital.

I came on to shift and had a 38-year-old that had been intubated. He had no medical history and had come in by ems after he collapsed at home. He had COVID and blood clots. I talked to his wife on the phone, and she stated he got the COVID shot two days prior and had been short of breath since. I told the doctor, and she said, "it looks like he got the shot too late." This was the response of the medical provider providing his care; it made me angry and sick. This man died a few days later, probably labeled unvaccinated death because it was not 14 days out of his second shot; it was 5 days after his first.

I came on to shift and had a very sick man; he had COVID and was on BiPAP. His wife was there with him, and she was tearful. I talked to her and him and asked her what happened to get him to this point. She said she didn't know he had both shots and wasn't supposed to be sick. I stood there wanting to scream, but the shots did nothing!! But I listened. I went out and looked at the computer; he had been there the whole day in the ER. He had an echo done; it showed that he had some strain on his heart and high pressures in his lungs. As I sat there, I listened to the off going doctor report to the oncoming doctor. He was talking about another patient that was there on oxygen; he snickered and said, "and he is not vaccinated." I snapped; I looked at him and said, well, what about the one in there? Who is doing worse and IS vaccinated? He quickly said, "well, he doesn't have his booster."

I knew my face became red in anger, and I just got up and walked away. This patient's wife was crying; I went back to the room and cried with her. I prayed with her. She pulled out awards and showed me that he was a veteran. He fought in the Gorilla wars and won awards. They were in the process of getting US veterans benefits but hadn't yet, and could I please help? I called the transfer center; I pleaded to get this guy transferred. I relayed that he was a hero and did what he was supposed to do and is now dying. Nothing was done.

    I went to the doctor and asked if he could give him vitamins, Ivermectin, and sildenafil. That he needed them to survive, he laughed at me and said he would get in trouble for providing these. Instead, the patient got admitted. I came back the next week, and he was still there. I went upstairs, and he was intubated and prone. After speaking with his wife, she told me about their four children, that all her family was in another country, and how she didn't know what she would do if he didn't make it. They had given him remdesivir and other medicine, and nothing was working. I again cried with her, prayed with her, and told her I would continue praying for her and him. Fast forward one more week, and when I returned, I was informed that he had passed away. I didn't get to see the wife again.

I got to work, and it was a mess, all the rooms were full, and someone was checking in with a headache. Yes, we all get headaches; in their defense, some get migraines that they can not control at home. So I brought her back, a young woman in her mid-forties, to triage her. As she started talking, it just sounded weird. She said, "I get migraines, but this is different." "Different, how," I asked. She said, "this will sound weird, but It hurt here, and then here, and then over here." She said it was over multiple days but pointed to different spots on her head. I looked at her and asked about her medical history and if she had the covid shot. She said, "well, ya, but that was a while ago." I said ok and that someone would be with her soon. I told doc her 'weird' story, and of course, he ordered a head CT, labs, and the 'migraine cocktail.' About 2hr later, I was stunned by the CT results; this woman, for every spot she had pointed to, about 5, had small brain bleeds. We had never seen anything like that, brain bleeds, small ones, in multiple spots on the brain. Guess it's another 'weird new thing' to get used to.

I came on to shift and had an elderly patient, 77 years old. He had bilateral pneumonia, was positive for Covid, and had to place on BiPAP. I went in to check on him; his wife sat next to him, asking why he had Covid when he had already gotten two shots. I thought to myself, do these people believe these shots work? I looked at her, smiled, and said, "it doesn't seem to matter." She seemed shocked but also accepted this; how could she not? Her husband struggled to breathe, and they knew he had two shots.

As I walked into work this night, I knew it would be nuts. There were stretchers in the hallways full and bells ringing. I walked into my first patient's room to introduce myself and ask why he was there. He said, "well, I got the booster, and now I have weird feelings. I am throwing up, and it's miserable." I asked why he got the booster; he said my job required it, and I had no problem with the first two. I relayed this to the doctor; he said it was normal. In my head, I know that neurological issues with throwing up after a medication is an adverse event. I would not give a patient medication to make them feel like this. It's weird how the medical providers now blindly dismiss these patients. He was discharged with a follow-up and Zofran.

During that same shift, our hospital system had a 21-year-old male with a stroke and a 28-year-old male with seizures. This is crazy. I went in to see my 28-year-old that had a seizure, who was now alert and vitals stable. He worked at a gas station and was able to get the recording of what happened to him because he didn't even realize what had happened. He showed me. As I watched this video, a young, healthy guy working falls straight down stiff, starts jerking violently, and then goes limp as another coworker comes rushing to him and calls 911. This makes me think of the videos from China, which have recordings of vaccine reactions of people having seizures. I asked this young man if he was vaccinated for COVID he said, "well, ya why" I said well, you need to report it to VAERS, I explained what that was, and he said he would. We discharged him.

This was not my patient, but in the ER, they are all my patients; there was a 15-year-old that came in. She was brought in having seizures. They were so bad the only way to control them was to sedate her and put a breathing tube in. She did not have a history of these; she was also vaccinated for COVID. It still astonishes me that people are not putting this together. I talked to a doctor that day; she said, "well, we have with teenagers and chest pain; we now do troponins on all ages." How is this just accepted as a new normal? A seven-year-old came in that evening with sharp chest pain and shortness of breath; yes, she was vaccinated, but they did no testing on her. I told the doctor there was an incidence of myocarditis with this shot, and he laughed and said, "you think everything is the shot." I said, "well, think back a couple of years; did you see this age group having chest pain?" He walked away.

Still traveling to the same small hospital, I see the death toll rise dramatically. When I started there, before they started giving out the vaccine, I don't think I had one code blue for the first 4 months. Then COVID and vaccine-related issues began flooding in the door. I had an intubated patient every shift for two months straight. I felt more like an ICU nurse for those two months than I did an ER nurse. We couldn't send them anywhere because all the hospitals were full. We were sending patients to Virginia if they even got beds at all.

Now the death rate has become crazy. Every shift I come in to, a code is either happening or has happened. One weekend there was a cumulative 4 cardiac arrests, ages 75, 52, 35, and 40. This was what I walked into. About an hour after being at work, thankfully, for the moment, the waiting room was empty. I think this was more Gods doing. We had a truck pull up, and he said he needed help with his wife. We walked out to the car, and she was laying over, blue, not breathing. She had no pulse. The man, her husband, said they had a 10-minute drive. So she had already been gone for that long; the doctor asked if he wanted us to do everything, and he said yes. We had nowhere to take this lady. All the rooms and hallways were full. We placed this lady on a stretcher. I jumped on the stretcher and started compressions. We walked in the front door, with me on the stretcher, and worked this code in the waiting room. We did our best, but we were not getting her back still. About 10 minutes into this, her daughters show up. They were upset and crying. We stopped the code a few minutes later, still in the waiting room we cleaned up. We finally got one patient out of a room and put her in there. She was vaccinated and had no cause of death.

That same weekend there were another 35-year-old and 49-year-old cardiac arrests. They also did not make it. The doctor says, "there are so many lately" I don't even know what to say anymore. How do you continuously tell these people, who are supposed to be so bright, what the reality is? It is like a merry-go-round that I am stuck on. One nurse got the covid shots, he used to run 5 miles, but he couldn't run for months. He is now getting to where he can get a little but has arthritic pain all over. I tried to convince a doctor that these shots were doing bad things by making him tell him his story; maybe since it's a nurse, he would listen; he said, "Oh, come on now." Jesus, I am getting more depressed by the day.

Another 3 shifts back, over this course of shifts, 10 cardiac arrests. WHAT IS GOING ON??!! Ages 53, 85, 24, 79, 74, 76, 60, 76, 50, 66; what is that average age? 64 is the average age of the death toll that happened over this 72hr period. How is this even possible? So we all agree that we live in the United States of America. We all agree that we are supposed to be the smartest and best country. Then why is it that the main medical establishment cant sees this? Has the perception of reality shifted, accompanied by the perception of good health and good healthcare? This is crazy. I walk in to work now with utter confusion, sadness, and horror. I am ashamed to be in healthcare at times. And then I pray and feel I am still where God wants me, but I am not sure I like it.

My Own Eyes

I came on to shift and went to discharge my patient in the hallway. She was an older lady in her 60s, so she was not that old. I read the instructions as I printed them, ovarian cancer. I asked the doctor her story before I went to discharge her. He said, "well, she has a huge mass, and it has metastasized to her bones." I asked well did you tell her? He said, "I told her she had some mass and will have to see oncology; she understands." I said, well, ya, but did you tell her how bad it was, he said, "that's not my job in the ER." UGH. I went to discharge this lady; she asked, "how am I supposed to get to my appointment?" I said well, you would have to get with social services. She asked about the pain she was having, and I said, "the doctor wrote you a prescription" she said ok and slowly made her way out the door. The next shift, I had an EMS come in, someone with back pain. It was her. This poor lady was suffering. Thank god I had a new doctor. I went to her and explained the patient's story. She said, "Oh my gosh, she needs hospice and pain control." Yes, this vaccinated lady, diagnosed with stage 4 ovarian cancer in her bones 2 days ago, needs hospice. This is the reality everyone is dismissing.

It was about 1 hour before leaving time. Overhead "CODE APGAR," this is a code no one ever wants to hear. An APGAR, activity, pulse, grimace, appearance, and respiration should be around 7-10. These scores are done at minutes one and five of a newborn's life. This newborn had an APGAR of 3 at one minute and five at five minutes. The mom had 3 shots while she was pregnant. She thought it would make her and the baby healthier and safer. This is not the case. This newborn got transferred and diagnosed with pulmonary hypertension. This means that a newborn with a full life ahead now has a chronic disability of high blood pressure in his lungs. This leads to heart failure and will shorten his life, if not kill him soon.

As I am getting ready for another shift, I am looking over the board to assess how the day has gone and what I have going on. I see that today there have been 2 cardiac arrests (68yo, 45yo) and a 3-year-old that had seizures and went to PICU. I know they had to intubate a 36-year-old, but I am not sure why. There was a 59 yo with altered mental status and a 38yo with a headache and heart rate of 141. This is a new trend I have seen, #1 younger cardiac arrests, #2 high blood pressure in all ages after the vaccine, and #3 lots of new AFIB and SVT. This trend continues the few days I am working. We have a 56-year-old male that's septic and a 27 yo male with a blood pressure of 64/42. Over the next few days, we have 3 more cardiac arrests, ages 76, 81, and 72.

Along with all the arrests and very sick people, I get a 19-year-old male that comes in with his mom. The story is that she found him in the bathroom unresponsive. She said, "he was blue; I had to do CPR." EMS was called to the house, she says, and they resuscitated him with Narcan. I start talking to him; other than looking very scared, he looks ok. I asked him, what did you take? He responds, "I took one Percocet, but I have taken more than that at a time, and nothing like this has happened." Mom says he is fine and just had his yearly check-up at the doctor's. She says, "he got his first covid shot today too." I stopped and looked at her. I asked, "he got a covid vaccine today," and she said, "well, ya at his doctor's appt." I walk out and tell the doctor; he rolls his eyes and says, " The kid took too many pills, and you think it's the shot. Well, I guess I am wrong again, ugh. I told myself to watch for him about 3 weeks later; if he goes and gets another shot, I pray he doesn't.

My next patient was a 65yo male with shortness of breath. His oxygen saturation was 74 on room air; he was struggling. I placed him on a non-rebreather at 15 liters and called respiratory and the doc to the room. We did the whole septic workup and sent him for a chest CT. He tested negative for COVID and was glad for that because he was vaccinated and boosted; his CT showed diffuse bilateral ground-glass opacities, which is the hallmark of covid-19. Still, at least he tested negative for it, right? I can't get over how this keeps going; even the doctors and about 90 percent of the nurses can't or don't see it. It's getting so absurd.

Today, this patient is probably the hardest I have ever had. I am not sure of the vaccination status of the mom/dad or patient. This situation punched me in the gut on how the healthcare system is collapsing, how incompetent care is increasing and being accepted, and how "good" healthcare professionals are getting wrapped up in horrible situations. I went out to get the newest patient that checked in. He was less than two months old. His mom brought him into the room in the car seat. I said let's take him out and started asking her questions. She said he had seen his pediatrician about 5 days ago and was diagnosed with RSV. She said he hadn't eaten much since then, had not pooped in a week, and his last wet diaper was in the morning, this was about 5 pm. I took him out of the car seat; he was lethargic and cold. I had another nurse in the room, and we put him on the pulse ox and took a rectal temp; it was 93.6. This made my heart sink; he was very sick. The mom continued to say he was born at 30 weeks, spent a month in NICU, and had only been home for 3 weeks.

I came out of the room to see who had signed up for this patient. I was ready to put in an IV, get labs, give fluids and sugar, and warm blankets. So I realized who it was and asked her to come to see the patient. After examining this patient, she said, "I think we will try skin-to-skin with mom and feed him." I looked at her in astonishment. I said, "this baby is sick; he needs a septic work-up," She said, "well, let's try this first." I wasn't happy; I got warm blankets, wrapped him and mom up, and talked to another doctor. He came and saw the baby and walked out and said, "ya, he doesn't look good" I said, "ok, can I get an IV now and treat him" he said, "ya," So I get the other nurse that was helping me, and we get all the

My Own Eyes

supplies to stick him, then the first doctor says, can you get his temp again. I am amazed that she thinks the past five minutes have fixed this baby. We do, and it's 94, still septic and bad. As we get the IV, this baby seems very lethargic; he barely cries. We wrap his arm where the IV is, and he goes apneic; his heart rate drops from 135 to 86, which is very low for a newborn. I sit him up, give him oxygen, and stimulate him by rubbing his back. Trying not to freak in front of the mom. I call the doc in, and she listens to his heart and verifies that his rate is that low; I call the other doc in. By this time, I had stimulated him, his heart rate was 130s again, and he was awake some. The doc walked in and said, "oh, he looks ok," I walked out behind him and said, "hey, his heart rate dropped, and he went apneic; this kid is going to crash." He walked away.

We get all the labs and urine and again have a mom in the bed with him, skin to skin, with warm blankets. But I am not walking out of the room. I just knew something was coming for this poor sweet one. So, about 5 minutes pass, he goes apneic, and his heart rate drops to the 80s. I walk over and stimulate him again, calling for help. At this point, I make it very clear. I asked one staff member to get the pediatric code cart, one to get oxygen, and one to put him on the crash cart monitor and be prepared for a code. At this point, I got the baby off of mom, the mom in the chair, and the baby placed on all monitors. He goes apneic, his heart rate drops, and someone starts compressions and bagging him. His heart rate comes up, and he responds.

In the interim of all this, the first doctor says, "I ordered a fluid bolus and antibiotics" She insists that he needs them right away. And though I agree with her that he needs them, I look at her with questions. He is getting bagged and compressions; antibiotics are not the cure ~~for me~~. But someone calls the pharmacy and makes sure that it's being prepared. Someone else calls down two pediatric nurses and a pediatrician. We put the patient in the baby warmer and cranked the heat, and I wish I had done that earlier. Still, the baby goes apneic, the heart rate goes down, and compressions again. Now they decide they will intubate him. The nurse with the crash cart asks for his weight and starts to pull out meds to medicate him. The doctor doesn't ask for meds; he asks for a tube. He attempts intubation and doesn't get it. They bag him. I finally asked when we would get this baby to another hospital with NICU and PICU; the first doctor said, "I made him an emergency so soon." The other doctor tries to intubate again, not successful. Then the pediatrician tries, then the respiratory therapist tries, and she says, "his airway is so swollen" I think it's because they have traumatized it.

After multiple attempts at intubation, they finally realized they wouldn't be successful. So now, the respiratory therapist uses an Ambu bag to keep him going. The transfer team gets to the room to fly him to another hospital, and they decide he needs to be intubated before flying. Here we go again. At least this team gives him some medicine to ease his pain. So they give him meds and attempt intubation, but it is no good. Try again; they get it, but it clogs with mucous, and they remove it. Then they bag for a little while, talking about what to do. They decide to try again, success. Finally, he has an airway; he got his antibiotics and fluids and was warmed up; now, please fly him to the PICU and get him the care he deserves. So they put him on a stretcher and brought him to the other hospital.

Later I found out that they lost his airway again on the flight and had to bag him to the hospital. He was intubated by intensive care, sedated, and still living last I knew. After he flew off, the first doctor came to me and said, "Hey, I want you to know you were right and I was wrong" I couldn't even respond. I just looked at her and said, "well, he is going now." The next day a nursing supervisor said: "hey, I want you to know that you did great charting, and all the 'big wigs' are looking into this because it is obvious it was physician, not nursing." "That is good because it was horrible care and an absolute shit show." She seemed surprised by my response, but who am I here to please? However, I looked up and was working with the same doctor again, so now I know how that goes. A huge screw-up that was not an accident but complete incompetence, and here she is to work another shift.

That was a horrible shift and the worst pediatric code I have ever been involved in. Sadly other nurses were traumatized by this incident as well. There was no debrief to air this; there was no "big wig" that talked to me and asked me questions. There was just the sly push-under-the-rug mentality that healthcare has become. It's so depressing; as hard as I try to yell it from the roof tops and protect patients, it's still a scary environment.

The next few days at work were not as bad as that day, but we were pretty busy with, yep, you guessed it, more obvious shot injuries. We had a 38-year-old who started having headaches a few days earlier and falling. His mom tried to get him to the hospital, but he wouldn't. Well, she finally convinced him, and guess what? This healthy 38-year-old had a right hemispheric hemorrhage with an 11mm right to left shift. This means he had a huge bleed, it was pushing on his brain, and he had to be transferred emergently to a neurologist. He was vaccinated about 1 year previous; I didn't ask about a booster. We had two other strokes on the same day. Also, both with vaccinations, but no medical establishment is putting these things together. Lord, why didn't I pick another career?

When all this madness of COVID started, as a healthcare professional, I couldn't understand why more people were not investigating the actual mechanism of action of the virus and drugs. I started getting interested in this fact and started investigating lab values. Of those who had COVID, of those who had been vaccinated with mRNA or johnsona and johnson, and those, like me, who had been exposed to vaccination and had covid. It was interesting to see

My Own Eyes

the trends, and now I can see them. By looking at an ED board, I can usually tell who is vaccinated most likely and who has COVID by looking at lab values.

One trend is blood pressure in the vaccinated is about 75% percent population elevated, even at young ages. In children, you are even seeing high blood pressure; in adults, it's uncontrollable. It's crazy how nurses and doctors alike have accepted very high blood pressure in patients. Before Covid, we never would discharge a patient with blood pressure over 180 systolic or 90 diastolic. The top number should be lower than 180, the normal is 120, and the high used to be considered 140. Now we have patients walking in with lacerations, with blood pressures over 200. And they say, "ya, it's been like that," so in the chart, it's written 'asymptomatic,' and we discharge. Another thing changing rapidly in healthcare is ignoring and accepting unhealthy patients and portraying them as the 'new norm.'

Another big one is new-onset diabetes with vaccination and having recently had COVID. The sad thing is, with early treatment, these kids would not get this new onset juvenile diabetes. I had a 7-year-old. Came in with abdominal pain and throwing up. He looked very 'puny,' which is the word I would use. His color was off, so I started an IV, and we got labs. For most kids, if they present with certain complaints, we start an IV and do a cat scan to check for appendicitis. This kid didn't appear appendicitis, but you never know. CT came back clear, but his labs didn't. His labs showed he was acidotic, and his glucose was high. His parents said he had never been sick before but had COVID recently. I then researched this, and some data showed that kids with recent covid were getting new-onset juvenile diabetes. I presented this to the doctor. He looked at me like I was crazy but accepted that his labs offered like it. We admitted the kid, and he was sent off to another hospital, so I did not get to follow up, the worst part about being an ER nurse. But now my eyes were open to another Covid-created issue with children.

When I came on to shift, I was worried about the approved new "bivalent" booster and what would happen now. Of course, I got the inside scoop from other nurses on what I had missed. In 72 hours, the deaths were eight. Eight people died in the ER in 72 hours. This does not include out-of-hospital deaths; I had talked to many EMS who said they were dropping everywhere. This does not include hospital deaths; all this is ER deaths. The ages of the deceased make it even worse, 37, 76, 64, 90, 91, 63, 26, 41. Do you know what makes the average age for dying these last 72 hours 60.875 or 61 years old? How is this not mind-blowing? This is two ERs in one small area; how many hospitals nationwide and worldwide are seeing this? How can this be ok? Where are the autopsies and data on why so many people are dying? Another sad day for healthcare.

I had a patient that came in with constipation. She was older,

My Own Eyes

about 75. Nice lady. I asked her when it started; she said, "well, they gave me some pain medicine after my biopsies." I wondered what biopsies she had done; she responded that she had to have biopsies on her kidneys and breast. She stated she had also gotten the new bivalent booster and was proud of it. I didn't even look when she proudly pulled out her vaccination card, made just for Convid, mind you, with 8 spots allowed. So I guess she isn't done with shooting up.

Anyways, the doctor ordered a stool softener and an enema. I wouldn't say I like enemas. I went back in, and the patient said, I just went to the bathroom finally and could have a large bowel movement. I was relieved; that meant I didn't have to do an enema. I told the doctor, and she said great, I will discharge her. I told her the patient's blood pressure was 251/122. She didn't even bat an eye; she asked, "does she feel ok?" I said, yes, she seems fine. So we discharged her with that blood pressure. This patient said, "oh, it's been like that for a while" is this not crazy? Sometimes I feel like I am crazy, wanting to understand how things that used to scream abnormal are now all ok and acceptable. Ugh, maybe I should have started a landscaping business.

In the last 72hr the ages of cardiac arrest in the ER do not include the field in the hospital; remember, these are just from two small hospital emergency rooms. So there were eight total, the ages 37, 76, 64, 90, 91, 63, 26, and 41. When you look at these ages, it should scream outrage. It should tell us something is wrong here, but no one says anything. They keep on going like its all normal. The average age now for this group is 61. When I started this, the average age was above 80, so what has changed? I watch certain doctors, obviously not the mainstream ones, and they are presenting facts from all over the world that the excess death is increasing. None of them have the statistics with age groups yet; it seems the government and health agencies aren't doing them; that's weird. But if you open your eyes, it's clear. I was talking to a nurse about this the other day, and she said if you see it through our lens, you can see what is happening, but you can't get others to see.

    I had another argument with a doctor. It started this time because he was talking about "studies" and how ivermectin DID NOT; yes, he said it is a matter of fact, it DID NOT WORK. I asked him where he got his knowledge from. I said, ok, you say no studies, but there have been so many they won't publish them. I asked him to research Uttar Pradesh and their medical packs they handed out. It was ivermectin, doxycycline, zpack, vitamins, and Tylenol. Things that cost pennies, and they had huge success. I asked him if he thought big pharma was a problem, and he agreed and said, "obviously" I said, why do you think they push medicines that they proclaim work but cost so much? He said, "that has nothing to do with it." I laughed because, again, he would not listen to reason. I can say that I feel I am slowly getting some PAs and MDs to hear.

And even if they don't agree yet, they are asking questions.

This weekend, I talked to another; he has always called me the crazy ivermectin nurse. This is his way of making fun of me without being mean. I am ok with that. It is funny, we were talking, and we figured out that I am only 3 days older than him; oddly, we disagreed so much, but I made it clear he should respect his elders, and we laughed. I was leaving my shift, and he stopped me, and we began talking again about ivermectin. I said I had used it on myself, my husband, and my two youngest kids; he said "how did it go" my husband returned after hiking, and his hands and feet were cold. He ran the vehicle into the front of the camper when he returned because he was so out of it. I gave him the higher dose, 0.6mg/kg, and some vitamins, and he felt fine within three hours. I threatened him for the next four days, but he finished the course. I also said that I still take it prophylactically, and of course, I couldn't get that many pills, so I took the horse paste. He laughed and said see horse med. I said that's cool, but I have used it every week for a year and a half, and I have stayed well. Without n95, without fear, and without getting ill. His eyes lit up; he said, "well, how much do you take?" I explained how the dosing was hard, and I had done it differently to figure it out, and that I now take about a fingertip and swallow it with water. The apple is not what I would call yummy, LOL. He just said, "oh, ok," it's funny how he makes fun of me but wants to know what I am doing and how. He then said he had signed his son up to get his vaccine; I sighed. I looked at him and said, "please think hard on that; please pray about it" he said, "ya," I said, especially in young men, there were vast cases of myocarditis, and it inflames the heart regardless of if its bad enough for him to realize. He just looked at me and nodded. He will probably get the shot; I pray he will be ok.

The next day I had a husband and wife come in. He was 98, and she was 90. Their daughter was with them. They both had Covid; the wife said, "we got 4 shots already, but we didn't get the new one; I guess we should have." I don't even know how to respond to this anymore. This woman, who has lived 90 years on this earth, is gullible enough to think that this virus that four shots haven't stopped would have magically been destroyed by a fifth and that this was their fault, not the fault of the pharma company that is selling a horrible product worldwide. How does this make sense in people's heads? I left the husband in the wheelchair and put the wife in the bed because I had brought them to one room. When I took their vitals, I realized the husband needed the bed; his blood pressure was very low. So we switched them and started an IV on the husband to bring his blood pressure up and get him some antibiotics. See, if it were just Covid, we would have done nothing, like for the wife. But because his blood pressure was low, he was lucky, rang the sepsis bell, and got fluids and antibiotics. Crazy how two years into this, we still don't treat covid at all. If the test says positive, we act like there is nothing to do.

I had two teenagers this shift. One of them was a young female; she had tics. When they were diagnosed, she said, "oh, about a year ago," I asked her and her dad if she had gotten the covid vaccine, and she said, "ya, like over a year ago" They looked at me like I was crazy. This girl was hitting herself in the face. Her tics were so bad; the dad looked on like this was not scary for his daughter, yet I was the crazy one. I then had a young man. He and his dad were so nice. He said, "well, I go to the gym every day, and usually, I have no issues" he continued, "I went yesterday, and my arms and legs were just weak, and they draw up like this." He shows me how his hands and legs start drawing up and getting tight, and he can't use them. It sounded like maybe an electrolyte problem, but it seemed odd. We did labs and did a scan, but everything came back normal. We gave him muscle relaxers and sent him home with no answers.

Five deaths this 72hr period, 82, 62, 61, 21, 62, and this is 72 hours. This is not a week; this is not even four days; it's 3 out of 7. Remember that. This makes the average age 57.6. Jesus, it is dropping every week. So when I hear the presented facts from other countries about the excess death worldwide, but they can not get the age ranges, I can see it's not the 70 and above that is increasing. It seems to keep getting lower and lower. I am utterly disgusted that not one CEO, CNO, or Medical director is saying anything. All the data I listen to and watch comes from the UK, Germany, Ireland, Africa, and Israel; it's always another country where I see the statistics of increased all-cause mortality.

Where is the CDC on this data? The CDC is a joke! Healthcare has become so political and biased that we are getting no facts or data in the United States. What is this? How do the CDC, FDA, WHO, CMS, JACHO, and ALL these organizations work? Any one of them could step up and say let's get the data and prove that we do not have this increased mortality here in the US, but they don't. They don't care or know it is happening and don't want to show it. I think, how could these scientists and doctors not see this? Walensky has five shots now, including the bivalent, and has COVID again after just having it and taking Paxlovid, which has shown to have rebound. They don't give an F; she is the dumbest person or the richest CDC director in history.

This week I had a 20-year-old that I treated two nights in a row. He came in because he got his COVID shot three days earlier. I asked him why he had done this; his mom said it was because he wanted a new job, and they required it. I am amazed that this is still happening. This kid is a healthy 20-year-old, and here was the government stepping in and forcing a shot that does nothing to stop this virus but does harm the person getting it. What exactly has healthcare become but an arm of governmental control, regardless of individual health and freedom? There is not even informed consent with this garbage. Suppose the person about to give him this shot had given true informed consent, they would say. In that case, This is a medication that will not stop you from getting or spreading this virus. It has side effects, including myocarditis, pericarditis, blood clots, tremors, tics, Guillain barre, tinnitus, bells palsy, heart attacks, seizures, prion disease, and sudden death. Do you think this kid would have produced his arm for the shot? And if he did, at least he would have been warned of the real effects (that are truly known).

The next night this same young man came in; he was worse. He looked pale and could not even walk to the bed. I hooked him up to the monitor, and his heart rate was not alarming, but I could tell he was not feeling well. I got an IV and gave some fluids. We gave him some medications to treat his dizziness and nausea. His mom was sitting there, and I asked again about his shot. I wondered if he was planning on getting the second one. His mom chimed in and said, "it didn't do this to me; I don't know why he is like this".

The kid said he wasn't going to get the second shot, but his mom seemed like she was in favor of it. What is wrong with this scenario? Any parent that sees their child reacting should not give or encourage more of it. They used to call that Munchausen's by proxy, where the parent purposely makes the child sick for attention. Now I don't think that is what is happening here; I think the mom sees that her son is being 'dramatic' because the rest of the family got the shot and had no problems. However, these were actual physical side effects; knowing what I do, the second one would be worse for him. I pray he makes the right decision and his mom supports that. I am a "live let live" kind of person and have tried to relax on educating everyone on this horrible medication, but it's also my job as a nurse educator. It's such a fine line.

This week, this 72hr, wow, is all I can say. Deaths 70, 67, 73, 62, 41, 48, 45, 55, 66, 5, 79, and 55. That is 12 deaths in 72 hours that I can see. How is this not huge? Yes, you read those ages right; this week, it includes a 5-year-old. There was also a 14-year-old with a heart rate of 155 and respiratory difficulty that came close. This may seem a little weird, but add those up, and your total is 666. How is that for a whole, and the average age is 55.5? Lower and lower we go.

My gosh, I want to scream. I turn to another nurse, one I can freely talk to, and say, do you see this? She gets a grim look and says, "yes, it's so obvious." How is this so obvious that more nurses are seeing it, but it's not apparent enough for healthcare to call it what it is? This shot is becoming a death and harmful event for everyone who participated. It causes a side effect, lowers your response, and makes an underlying condition more lethal. Ugh, sometimes I see those clown emojis in my head when I talk to some healthcare workers. I have had daily arguments about increased all-cause mortality and increased death in younger and younger patients.

My Own Eyes

Along my journey of discovery, big pharma and the push on these shots have opened my eyes to other images. And this, to me, is heartbreaking. Childhood vaccines, I have always been a clear fan of. From a healthcare standpoint, historically, how vaccines were made all made sense to me. Scientifically you introduce a dead piece or abstract piece of a virus, and your body reacts to it, creating the antibodies needed. Here is the part I missed, to get your body to react strongly enough, big pharma companies added harmful by-products to the viral particle. This means they found the most poisonous chemical or solution, added it to the viral particle, and then got a higher antibody response. Now I will have to study this more, of course, and I am not saying this as a vaccine researcher, merely a nurse educator who sees things differently. One has five kids who all have their childhood vaccines, and I wish I had researched this earlier and not had them. I would say my kids did not get autism as some do. However, my oldest got an ear infection terrible, and every time she had an appt to get shots, about a week later, we were back or in the ER for temps of 105 and an ear infection. I always blamed breastfeeding in bed or her being sensitive to them; I never correlated

My youngest started with respiratory issues very early. She got pneumonia very young, was about 1, and her temp was so high the urgent care was scared to see her. She gets ear infections frequently, and when she got Covid, she was sick and got pneumonia. I fought to get her antibiotics because they labeled covid and ignored them. I also used ivermectin with her, and every time I stopped using it, she got sick again. So she took it for a very long time. She then got an ear infection which led to bells palsy, which the urgent care would not see her for and made us go to the ER. She also has been allergy tested because she started having reactions to many things, and now has a list of over 20 things she can not eat. It is crazy how these vaccines can taint the system and mess with the immune system. You ask why it was always urgent care; I stopped taking my kids to pediatricians right after I had my youngest. Every time we went, they wanted to give us another shot or another test. I was tired of constantly explaining that my kids were not getting more shots, were healthy, and didn't need a test all the time. And this was before Covid was even a thing. So it shocks me when parents get their young, healthy children a flu shot every year, and pediatricians push this.

  I had a five-year-old that came in this weekend; he had a fever. When I brought him back and started talking to his mom, asking what led up to this, she said, "He got his flu shot on Thursday, and that night, he had a seizure and fever." She then said that it was three days ago, and he still had high fevers. I looked at this poor kid, who had rosy cheeks and didn't seem like he felt good. His temp was 104. When the doc came and saw him, he was diagnosed with a left ear infection and placed on antibiotics. This takes me back to my oldest, who always got ear infections after her shots. It made me question why the mom had gotten him ~~for~~ a flu shot; she said, "I don't know what the doctor said he needed." Its sad how many young parents, including me, got shots for their children without saying why or the rationale. Now I can say that being in healthcare now, I know and always ask, but my oldest is 22; it's not like at 18, I had this knowledge. I assumed the doctor did know and trusted that.

This week was full of RSV and flu. The season has begun, and we have a lot of kiddos. I always see a rise at this time of year, but it seems worse this year. CDC says it's because kids need an RSV vaccine. Are you kidding me? They have tried this before, and it was stopped for ADE and failure. Please, any parents out there, research before getting this. That is one thing I know for sure, the difference between RNA and DNA viruses. They have to change the flu shot every year because the virus is RNA and mutates constantly. That is the same with Covid; that is why the shots don't work.

Along with other reasons, the scientific basis is that when they modify the covid shot, its to the current strain and then comes out when another strain is current. That is the simple way of putting it. No, no, kids, nor older adults, need a shot for RSV. We need to realize that when we locked down for Covid, many of these kids were inside a lot. They were not exposed to normal viral particles in society, like the 'bubble kid'; they were all hidden from the germs that create a healthy immune system. They were also masked, which caused worse lung and respiratory responses. So you have kids that weren't exposed, unhealthy lungs and respiratory tracts, and baam, you have an unprecedented RSV and Flu season. Scientifically, this makes sense; all kids need are some vitamins, sunshine, and fresh air. God gave them everything else.

This 72hr seemed a little calmer, 59, 79, and 86. So three deaths, average age 74.6, so at least a little higher than what it has been. But then I looked again, sadly, a 5-week-old. Jesus, this takes it back down to 56. I was talking to a paramedic, and she said that her 22-year-old friend had just started in the police force locally. She said he was already about to quit. I asked why, and she said he was the first to respond to a 5month old and 8-month-old cardiac arrests, and they both died. This had taken a huge toll on him psychologically, I can imagine. So as you can see, the ones I get are far from what is happening in society and inside the hospital. Remember, this is a small place, one city in one state; how many die there, and when will this be acknowledged?

So, this is becoming the norm now that vaccinated and boosted older adults are dying. We had an 80-year-old that was dying of Covid. Her whole family was in the room and was very attentive. At one point, they asked why we were not doing more for her, she was on BiPAP, but she had clear instructions she was not to be intubated or resuscitated. We told this family member that, and

My Own Eyes

he said, "well, that was her wish" we said well, we have to respect that. He then started saying that it was the fault of the nursing staff, the ones that didn't have their vaccine. This always raises the hairs on my neck. It's a mix of feeling ashamed for them saying I am in the wrong, angry at the accusation I have caused, and sad that they believe this. Another nurse chimed in and said, "wait, isn't your family member vaccinated?" he said, "well yeah." She said didn't she get a booster; he said, "she had two." The nurse then says, so how on God's green earth do you think that us having a vaccine would stop her from getting or dying from Covid when she had four shots? He couldn't answer this because it made no sense. But this is the daily bashing the unvaccinated healthcare workers get. I am used to it, but the emotions run through me every time. My husband always says, "stop caring about that," but he doesn't understand when you are constantly criticized and put down and accused of doing something wrong, you slowly get depressed, anxious, and angry. At least I do, but I am working on letting that go.

 I had another patient this week; he was young 20s, newly married, and he and his wife had Covid. He seemed sicker than average 20-year-olds with Covid; some with sore throats come in for a test and leave. But this one was pale and diaphoretic. His heart rate was 147, so I went ahead and started an IV and gave him fluids. As I was sitting there, he said how lucky he and his new wife had been because they hadn't gotten covid since the beginning. I said, "oh, that is lucky." He said we got vaccinated a while ago, and I guess I should have gotten that booster. I just stayed quiet. This young couple, starting in life, is so swayed by the current corrupt big pharma game that they think it's their fault for getting covid because they did not get "that new booster." When will people realize that constantly messing with your immune system and responses will only harm your natural defenses? If you keep altering the innate immune system's ability to fight, your immune system will lose its ability completely and rely solely on the outside (help), shots or medications. I hope one day I can leave the "system" and work where I can teach natural health and healing. This was another very healthy young man who had been jabbed with medication that didn't work and is now sick with the virus it was meant to protect from, and he blames himself. So sad makes me so sad.

We had an 80-year-old man; I wouldn't, in the past, always assume that the covid vaccine is the cause of everything, especially in the elderly. But I guess that is how it is supposed to work; the mRNA seeks out weakness in the host and expounds it. So this gentleman, the father of one of my coworkers, came in with a massive GI bleed. The ER and admitting MD assumed that he was a drinker. We see these bleeds with alcoholics because they usually ruin their liver and esophagus. So the doctor asked him. And he was shocked by the question; he said, "no, I am a preacher," so, the doctor's response, you ask? "It must have been all the preaching over the years." Are they serious? So now preachers can't talk, or they will have massive upper and lower gastrointestinal bleeding? I spoke to the daughter over the time he was with us, and she said, "daddy has been going down since he got that vaccine; I know that is what this is." This man, who has served God all his life, preached the word and followed "the science," now had to get multiple units of blood and rehab. Sadly I am sure this won't end for him, but thankfully he is a follower of Christ. It is sad to keep seeing this repetition and side effects that no one calls out. I sometimes truly feel I am in the twilight zone in healthcare.

More and more nurses are coming to me lately and saying they agree with me. It is slowly turning, I think. One nurse, who is also a traveler, is very open with me and has no problem speaking her mind about these shots. She told me that her dad recently had a heart attack, the second one since his shots. And she said when the cardiologist talked to her after his heart cath, he said the clot was "white platelets." WHAT?? I watched Dr. Cole, met him in Tennessee, and he does many pathology explanations behind these shots. As well as post-mortem exams of covid vaccine recipients, they have "white fibrous clots"; this isn't platelets or natural clotting. This same nurse, her aunt, died after getting her covid vaccine booster. How is this still happening, and how can we stop the madness?

Congestive heart failure is when your heart does not beat

strong enough to pump all the blood and fluid out of your body. When your heart can't beat strong enough to get that fluid, it gets caught in your legs and lungs. It's a challenging diagnosis and a lifelong commitment to eat right and drink the right amount to not have your heart fail more and not have the fluid build-up so you can't breathe. So we see this diagnosis frequently; it's not unusual. However, it has become more and more "sudden onset." I had an 86-year-old female that came in; she had just been diagnosed with congestive heart failure, she had gone to her doctors and was "doing what they told her to do." She had severe "pitting edema," which means swelling so bad when you push on it, it doesn't bounce back. It was in both her legs. So I asked her when it started, and she said, "Oh, a couple of days ago." Usually, when someone has this bad of swelling, they have an abnormal lab called BNP. Hers was normal, so you have someone doing all the right things, no abnormal labs, but her symptoms are obvious. This is also becoming quite frequent with vaccine recipients. They come in with severe complaints, everything lab-wise and scan-wise looks normal, so they are either made to feel they are faking it or that nothing is wrong, and they can go home and deal with it.

This week the age range is so much lower; ugh, it is so sad. 46, 46, 69, and 13. This makes only four. However, the average age is 43.5!! Forty-three and a half is this week's average age of death. And these are just deaths I see in the ER; these are not at home, community, or in-hospital deaths. How crazy is this? When in history has this happened? How is this acceptable, and people keep going? I have been stressing over this for years; it seems like an eternity. And sometimes I think I will wake up and "they" finally announce that "they" are stopping these shots. That "they" were wrong. But it never happens, and I am slowly getting angrier and sadder by the day.

Tonight I had a 17-year-old. She was brought in by her dad, who works in healthcare. She was crying, and it was obvious she was in pain. She complained of abdominal pain. We thought it might be appendicitis, so we ran the labs and waited for her CT results. I learned she had been vaccinated, but that does not even surprise me anymore. Her labs came back; ugh, they looked bad. Just all over the place, but nothing specific that you could diagnose. Her CT came back; it was clean. No appendicitis, no gallbladder issue, and a normal abdomen. So many with labs and scans looking normal, the patient is obviously in distress; we drug, make them feel better for that moment and send them home. No answer, no real help, just a momentary fix; that's what we do now, fix the moment, not the patient.

Since last week, the deaths seemed to slow for a minute, and there wouldn't be as many this week. I was wrong; there were ten. 36, 45, 75, 66, 53, 67, 85, 76, 76, and 79. WOW, it seems it's not going to slow down yet, and the ER has been so busy lately. It is insane; this week's deaths average, 65.8, so about 66 years old. Not as bad as last week, but the average lifespan should not be this low. It is crazy how many sick people we have lately, too. Not just deaths, the flu, RSV, MPV, the least we have is covid. Also had a 28-year-old with a head bleed; I have never seen so many heads bleeds than in the last two years. Blood pressures are also still sky high in all vaccinated patients; I can almost pick out the ones of any age that have been vaccinated by looking at the vital signs on the board and seeing their blood pressure. It's unique and more impressive that doctors now accept these high blood pressures, not treat them as much because it's every patient.

Another week and again, how low the average age of death scares me. Only four ends, but 77, 49, 6 month old, and 25. That takes the average age down to 37.875!! That is younger than me!! Jesus helps us all. I truly believe in ten to fifteen years, this timeframe will be a very dark time in history. It will be construed in so many ways; that is one reason I am writing this book, to put some facts and truth that I have seen with my own eyes to the history that I am sure will be twisted.

You know, most people have this mentality with "shots" or "vaccines" in general: they get them to protect themselves and others. That is what we were all taught. I got my kids all their childhood vaccines; I thought I was doing the right thing. I was born in the 80s, so I didn't have as many as them, so when I went to nursing school and had to show proof I didn't have the varicella vaccine. I also didn't remember if I had chicken pox. So they said I had to get the vaccine; instead, I got the titer test. This will show if you have antibodies to something. I feel this is one educational piece to this scam of covid vaccines. But I think it's also with all the shots now. I had a 78-year-old gentleman that came in. He was weak, had fevers and congestion, and looked like the flu.

I talked to the daughter, and she said he started feeling weak two days after getting his "flu shot." I said well, it looks like the shot gave him ago the flu. She looked at me astounded like I had done or said something wrong. I simply walked out. We swabbed him with the regular flu/RSV/covid swabs. His flu swab came back positive. I didn't laugh at the fact that I was right, nor did I feel happy. Instead, I felt terrible for them. The father was sick as a septic dog, the daughter loved her dad and waited on him hand and foot, and the grandson called to facetime him to make him feel better. I did not even want to tell them it was the flu and he got it from the shot, but I did.

And interestingly and sadly enough, the daughter just said, "Ok, well, we knew it wasn't 100 percent". UGH, healthcare has become so dismantled and fragmented. People blindly accept and move on most of the time, don't question.

This week there were four, 25, 56, 53, and 57, making the

average age 47.75. Well, at least it's older than me, but barely. I had another patient in with swelling to her legs. We scale swelling, or edema, by numbers. One is up to 2mm when pushed and comes back up immediately. 2 is 3–4mm when pushed and comes back in 15 seconds or less. 3 is 5–6mm of down and comes back in 60 seconds. And 4 is 8mm indented when pushed and comes back very slow, usually 2–3 minutes. This lady had plus 3 pitting edema in her legs. She did not have congestive heart failure, her doctor put her on medication to help with this, but it was getting worse. It was so swollen it looked painful. So we checked her labs, and all was normal. She had high blood pressure, swollen legs, no answer, and four moderna shots. We keep moving forward, and people slowly fall apart, depend more on healthcare and less on themselves, and take whatever they are given.

It was a sad shift today; I had two cancer patients. Both of them, of course, didn't have COVID because they were vaccinated, which seems to matter most. But they were both losing their lives quickly. One was a charming 40-year-old woman. She was diagnosed with ovarian cancer last year, now in her lungs. There wasn't much to do; you can't save someone at this point. The other was an elderly gentleman who came in altered. We had him on BiPAP, and the family got there and was very upset. He was diagnosed with lung cancer last month, and they were already doing radiation treatment for it, so they were not sure what was happening.

My Own Eyes

We did scans, and the tumor in his lungs had shrunk a tiny bit, but it had spread like wildfire and was in his brain, causing swelling. UGH, the family was not ready for this diagnosis. No one ever is; they chose to keep him a full code and intubate him. Lord, I can not say I wouldn't have done this. But I am sure I would have had a good reason. I grew up in the system, so I can only relate to families making these scary decisions as if I were making it for one of my children. How can you let go? They were eating dinner together 6 hours before this. It's insane that we do this "for science," and "it's safe and effective," is all they hear. But now a family is losing a dad, a husband, and a good man because they, too, "did what they were supposed to do." Its so depressing.

We had a patient today that was in a very frustrating situation. He was 75, short of breath, septic, and had to be put on BiPAP. We, of course, had to do the usual swabs, RSV/flu/covid. He got very demanding and angry. He said, I have been fully vaccinated, and I don't see the point in all this; just fix me. I explained that the vaccine doesn't stop you from getting covid, it doesn't stop you from getting very sick with covid, and it doesn't stop you from dying with or from covid. He said I was oblivious and was wrong. I smiled, said ok, and swabbed him. His covid came back positive. Again, I don't feel happy at these moments I feel ashamed. He was ashamed to be in healthcare, a system that told this man it would protect him if he took a shot. That if he took this "vaccine," he would be spared. Instead, I had to go and tell him that he had covid, opacities in his lungs that looked like covid, and that he was struggling to breathe because of covid. Just the state of what healthcare is, it's not even shocking anymore.

Today I had a 14-year-old, sweet kid. He was in a lot of pain and could barely walk. I thought it was a testicular torsion and went and got the doctor. We did labs and ultrasounds and then had the answer. This kiddo had epididymitis and orchitis pyocele. This means he had swelling, infection, and inflammation with a possible abscess to his scrotum. This 14-year-old innocent kid had severe disease in his testicles, and the doctor was not even shocked. The family was not surprised. I WAS shocked. You hardly see this diagnosis in adults; I have never seen it in a child. Can it happen, yes? But all these "things" that I have never seen before have only occurred in the last couple of years. So we can assume all we want in and out of healthcare, but these shots are tearing down immune systems, making small pathogens and bugs take a bigger toll on people because they can't fight them.

I met a very interesting lady this weekend. Now I have been against these shots since day one. I have been to many places talking against them, handing out flyers, and following physicians and nurses against them, but I had never heard of this lady. She was a nurse. She told me she was a DON of a nursing facility. She loved her job and supported her staff and patients like any great nurse. She said when the shots came out, I was ok with it. She said she got an email from her " higher-ups" telling her she was respected and a leader and should do the right thing. She agreed and wanted to be that "great" leader. So she got a moderna shot. She said she immediately started having tremors, seizures, and pain. She said she was shunned. She reported it, but nothing happened. She spoke out, but nothing happened. She filed a report, but nothing happened. Now I am meeting this woman, who is having abdominal pain, and we can't find anything wrong. She says, "I am used to that" she has been told so many times over the last two years that nothing is wrong. This woman, a nurse, and a fantastic leader was stripped of her life after just one Moderna shot. Not only was she stripped of her life, but she was also told and still is told, "nothing is wrong." Her husband was there as well; he had put everything on hold to take care of her. She can't drive, she can't work, and she is disabled, but the state won't even approve her disability; yes, she is fighting for that. I talked with this woman for a long time; I hugged her and apologized. I didn't put that shot in her, but society did. Our healthcare did, and our government did. And she was now suffering a slow decline and would not recover. She said some treatments she has tried have worked, but she will never return to what she was. And it only took one shot; how many people have taken 1,2,3,4 or even five shots? So sad.

    71, 75, 61, 28, 79, and 59, the ages for this week. Making the average 62.167, going up, thank god but still so young for a middle-age span. I wonder when the US will catch up with their death rate and average life span and how it will shock people. This week we also had a 37-year-old with a stroke, a common trend.

One kiddo I had, came in saying his chest was hurting. But it was only sometimes. I asked if he had gotten the covid vaccine, and he said yes because he was going to fly to see his new girlfriend. His mom was excited for him. I said well, it sounds like you have pericarditis. It sounds similar to my daughter and what happened to her. They both looked at me. I said well, we would see; maybe it's nothing. So we did his EKG and labs. While waiting on the results, I got a call from the lab. A normal troponin is less than 0.03; they called with his result, which was 1.62. I can even; it's almost comical now when I argue with patients and doctors because I see what is happening and they still act shocked. So I tell the doctor, and he says, "welp looks like he needs an echo." This is an ultrasound of the heart. So, I explain the process, the echo, the cardiologist, and the medication to the mom and him. The kid asks, will I be able to see my girlfriend? This is the chaos we have created now. He wants to be fixed and move on. I didn't tell him my daughter is about 18 months out of it and still has issues. I guess I will leave that conversation for his next medical visit.

Today I walked in and walked by a room; it had a screaming baby and lots of beeping going on. I walked in. It was a 10month old. He was on high-flow oxygen. The mom looked exhausted, and he was not giving up. He did not like the oxygen on him, but he sounded horrible, and his oxygen would drop if he moved it. So I tried to calm him and mom down. I talked to the nurse caring for him and found out he had bronchiolitis. This is inflammation of the bronchioles and lungs, and breathing was hard. A virus usually causes it; low and behold, this kid was given the PCV13 vaccine two days previous. He had a well-baby visit and was given this shot. I admit, I got my children their childhood vaccines, but why on earth are we giving children pneumonia and flu shots? I never got those. I stopped taking my kids to pediatricians after the age of two, only because they were healthy, and I didn't want them to get those. So now we have this baby that is sick from a vaccine and has to be admitted to the hospital on oxygen, and we all go about the day.

Today, this patient made it clear that he had gotten 5 covid shots. I want to scream when patients stand tall and firm on the fact that they are protected from covid because of these shots. This patient had ground glass opacities on his lungs; this is what covid looks like. He also now had lymphoma, cancer, in his lymph node system. So as he boldly tells me he doesn't have COVID, I have to say that he does have cancer, sadly.

Chapter 04

Ending

It haunts me how many of these stories there are. I have many more. So many nurses and healthcare providers have many more. So, when I was in the hospital with my daughter in Nov of 2021, I joined telegram. I joined an Australian Christian healthcare workers group. I was sad to hear what was happening in Australia and wanted to pray for and with them. Instead, they prayed for my daughter and me. The few that I talked to were able to help me get through a horrible moment in my life. God led me there and to the patriot pages after that. So then I got involved in the NC pages and then the convoy. I volunteered and became the Care Package 81. I helped with donations for our group; never having done anything like this, I got a huge store full of care packages, donations, and even gift cards. I then adopted a trucker, as I thought everyone should be responsible for improving this situation. And I could not have gotten all the donations without the team we had; it was awesome!

As a nurse educator, I have been trying to educate those around me. The people I work with know me as the Psycho ivermectin nurse, my husband sometimes jokes and asks if I want a foil hat (he says with love), and my nurse counterparts have yelled at me. I wrote an educational letter that I started distributing to hospital staff. One morning as I was doing this (with another awesome nurse), a nurse started yelling at me. She said in no way was I a nurse, nor was I educated. She said I was spreading propaganda and should be ashamed. She asked security if they could remove me, I was on a public sidewalk, so they couldn't. Inside, my heart always sinks in these moments; I get embarrassed, question myself, and ask God if I am doing his work. But on the outside, I smiled while this nurse threw my letter back at me and jumped around because she was so angry. I said, "if you don't believe me, just research it," she said, "I don't have to; I have worked the last two years in it." I just said, well, have a good day.

This story has been what it has been like, for one simple nurse, in the last few years. Covid has affected everyone worldwide, and I don't think that any person in healthcare, in society, has had an easy time. I wrote this book because I wanted to put down in writing what truly is happening in the healthcare system with my own eyes. It is not something I am proud of; it depresses me and makes me scared of the future. I have researched enough to know that here in the United States, they keep early treatment away from patients; they are pushing "vaccines" that do not stop this virus and are unsafe. There is no risk-benefit scale. When done correctly, it would show that the benefits DO NOT outweigh the risk. There is no way anyone can truly say that the death toll from the shots, covid, and the aftermath of combining them has not increased all-cause mortality nor lowered the average age of death.

In writing this book, I hope to open some eyes and encourage others that have seen the same or experienced what I have to talk about it openly. To have the conversations. I feel that in the future, this time in history, if looked at honestly, will be very dark in history. I am also worried that it won't be looked at honestly, and this book is a way to prayfully shed some light on what will be kept in the dark. I also wrote this book as a type of therapy for myself. I feel, and I am sure there are nurses nationwide and worldwide, who feel so lost, worried, stressed, and even ashamed to be in healthcare. I want all healthcare and people that are not healthcare to see that there are still some of us who know what real healthcare is. I understand that what has happened over the last few years has been a failure. That some of us will walk away out of this fear, shame and stress. Still, I hope to encourage those medical professionals to stand up again and know that they are where God put them. Somehow we must mend this system again to be patient advocates, self-advocates, and co-worker advocates and see healthcare become a stronger and better thing for us all.